The Mediterranean Diet

Everything You Need to Know to Lose Weight and
Lower Your Risk of Heart Disease
with Delicious Recipes

(Everything you Need to Know to get Started)

Tamara Henderson

Published by Jason Thawne Publishing House

© Tamara Henderson

The Mediterranean Diet: Everything You Need To Know To Lose Weight And Lower Your Risk Of Heart Disease With Delicious Recipes

(Everything You Need To Know To Get Started)

All Rights Reserved

ISBN 978-1-989749-81-4

This document is geared towards providing exact and reliable information in regards to the topic and issue covered. The publication is sold with the idea that the publisher isn't required to render accounting, officially permitted, or otherwise, qualified services. If advice is necessary, legal or even professional, a practiced individual in the profession should be ordered.

- From a Declaration of Principles which was accepted and approved equally by a Committee of the American Bar Association and a Committee of Publishers and Associations.

In no way is it legal to reproduce, duplicate, or even transmit any part of this document in either electronic means or in printed format. Recording of this publication is strictly prohibited and any storage of this document isn't allowed unless with proper written permission from the publisher. All rights reserved.

The information provided herein is stated to be truthful and consistent, in that any liability, in terms of inattention or otherwise, by any usage or abuse of any policies, processes, or directions contained within is the solitary and also utter responsibility of the recipient reader. Under no circumstances will any legal responsibility or blame be held against the publisher for any reparation, damages, or monetary loss due to the information herein, either directly or indirectly.

Respective authors own all copyrights not held by the publisher.

The information herein is offered for just informational purposes solely, and is universal as so. The presentation of the information is without contract or any type of guarantee assurance.

The trademarks that are used are without any consent, and also the publication of the trademark is without permission or backing by the trademark owner. All trademarks and brands within this book are for clarifying purposes only and are the owned by the owners themselves, not affiliated with this document.

TABLE OF CONTENTS

Part 1 1

Introduction: 2

Meal Plan: 21

Pro Diet Tips: 26

Mediterranean Diet Recipes 46

Roasted Salmon With Black Pepper Sauce 46

Chicken Cheese In Roll 47

Mixed Vegetables Salads With Olive Dressing... 48

Asparagus Soup 49

Peanut Pancake With Maple Syrup 50

Choco Peanut Waffle 51

Carrot Tomato Omelets 51

Chicken Teriyaki... 52

Asian Beef Curry 53

Bacon And Cheese Scrambled Egg 55

Part 2... 57

Breakfast Recipes 58

Cookies With Peanut Butter............................. 58

Spinach Salad-Greek Version 59

Special Coleslaw 60

Paleo Pudding.. 61

Spinach Omelet 61

Hot Cereal 63

Fat Scramble.. 64

Tea Special.. 64

Burrito Breakfast Style 65

Banana And Cheese 66

Egg And Cheese Sandwich 67

Almond, Blueberries And Cheese...................... 68

Veggie Omelet 68

Protein Crepes 70

Broccoli Cheese Soup...................................... 71

Lime Cheese Cake 72

Asian Noodles.. 73

Scrambled Eggs... 74

Lunch Recipes 75

Lemon Chicken Soup....................................... 75

Beef Broccoli.. 76

Baked Chicken Thighs 77

Low Carb Meatballs 78

Chicken And Mushrooms 79

Slow Cooker Taco Soup................................... 80

- Slow Cooker Squash.. 81
- Fiesta Bean Dips 82
- Rib-Eye And Pepper 83
- Mexican Dip... 84
- Roasted Rack Of Lamb, Fennel, Cauliflower And Celery 85
- Sauted Greens And Poached Eggs..................... 86
- Salmon Avocado Lunch 86
- Sweet And Spicy Slow Cooker Chicken.............. 87
- Black Bean, Corn And Red Pepper Salad With Lime Cilantro Vinaigrette 88
- Corn Chowder... 90
- Dinner Recipes.. 91
- Roasted Pepper And Cauliflower 91
- Slow Cooker Buffalo Chicken Soup.................... 93
- Spaghetti Squash Lasagna................................. 94
- Cucumber Sandwich 96
- Borscht 96
- Minestrone... 98
- Lentil Soup.. 99
- Fried Eggs With Green Salsa.............................101
- Prosciutto-Wrapped Scallops...........................102

Spinach Stuffed Mushrooms 103

Salmon Fillet With Cucumber 105

Chicken Culets With Mustard............................106

Cauli-Tots 107

Roasted Cod With Butter And Garlic Lentil.......108

Quinoa And Smoked Tofu Salad 110

Baked Tortellini..112

Slow Cooker Chicken Dressing 113

Slow Cooker Buffalo Brisket..............................114

Slow Cooker White Chili 115

Main Dishes 116

Asparagus And Chipotle Mayonnaise...............117

Creamed Spinach...117

Chicken Curry 118

Ginger Beef...120

Chicken Salad...121

Beef Scramble And Egg Whites 122

Fried Chicken 123

Baked Salmon 124

Curried Pecans...126

Pecans 127

Conclusion 128
About The Author 128

Part 1

Introduction:

Congratulations for having this book!! This book provides a complete guidance of Mediterranean diet. Has been known as the healthy way in controlling weight and reducing the risk of having heart diseases, stroke, diabetes, cancer, and other chronic conditions, the Mediterranean diet is a dieting method that shows the way of eating in the countries at the boundaries of Mediterranean Sea. It is an effective dieting method that is easy to understand and follow. Having a pyramid of permitted food, Mediterranean diet concerns a lot on the food intake every person should have. This makes Mediterranean diet becomes a trusted dieting method to apply.

This book is completed with a comprehensive step-by-step guide and meal plan for those who want to apply the Mediterranean diet. This book offers 31 days of meal plans with tips and tricks to make the readers understand the book easier. Furthermore, this book also provides hints to kick off this dieting method with complete information. As Mediterranean territory is famous with delicious traditional cuisines, it is best to bring the menu to your dining table so that you will enjoy having the diet with appetizing cookeries. For that aim, this book also delivers a bunch of recipes that you can try. The recipes in this book are easy to cook with your simple equipment in the kitchen and become the best choices of menus, as they do not need a lot of time to prepare. So, save your time and grab this collection of recipes—from Roasted Salmon with Black Pepper Sauce, Chicken Cheese in Roll, Mixed Vegetables Salads with Olive Dressing, Asparagus Soup, Peanut Pancake with Maple Syrup, Choco Peanut Waffle to Chicken Teriyaki and many more! Bring the scrumptious meal from Mediterranean, enjoy your diet and be healthy!!

Day 1

Pro Diet Tips:
Before starting to apply the dieting method, it is best to know what Mediterranean diet is. Mediterranean diet is a dieting method that imitates the traditional healthy living habits of people who live in the countries at the boundary of the Mediterranean Sea. For centuries, the people in Mediterranean have been acknowledged as societies with exceptional health condition and fitness. Therefore, the lifestyles are accommodated into a dieting technique that can be applied by people worldwide.

Meal Plan:
Actually, applying Mediterranean diet is not difficult. However, diet is sometimes so challenging in the beginning. On the first day, it is suggested for you to still incorporated some meals, which are similar to your daily menu. The purpose is to make your body adapts to this new dieting method.

Breakfast	Lunch	Dinner	Snack

| Banana Pancake | Tuna and Vegetables Salads | Roasted Salmon with Black Pepper Sauce* | Steamed Carrot |

*The recipe is available in the last chapter of the book.

Day 2

Pro　　　　　Diet　　　　　Tips:
The Mediterranean diet is not just a fad of diet. Yet, it is a healthy way of eating with tons of benefits. Adopting the eating habits from ancient Mediterranean people who lived longer and disease free, Mediterranean diet is believed to reduce the risk of diabetes, heart diseases, stroke, Alzheimer, and other diseases. So, besides controlling your weight, Mediterranean diet helps you to increase your health condition　　　　　as　　　　　well.
Meal Plan:

From day 2, you will start to be more into the Mediterranean. You are going to start to have a meal plan that contains of the food approved by Mediterranean diet. For the second day, you will have a slice of toast with poached egg to start your brightly morning.

Breakfast	Lunch	Dinner	Snack
A slice of Toast with Strawberry Jam	Chicken Cheese in Roll*	Roasted Eggplant and Spicy Chicken	Piece of Fruit

*The recipe is available in the last chapter of the book.

Day 3
Pro Diet Tips:

Before you go further, you have to know what is the food to eat in Mediterranean diet and what to avoid. The aim of this knowledge is to make the right choice in picking the menu to support your diet. Some of the food might not be in your daily menu before, but keeping things simple will help you to adjust. This is the pyramid showing the food to be eaten in Mediterranean diet.

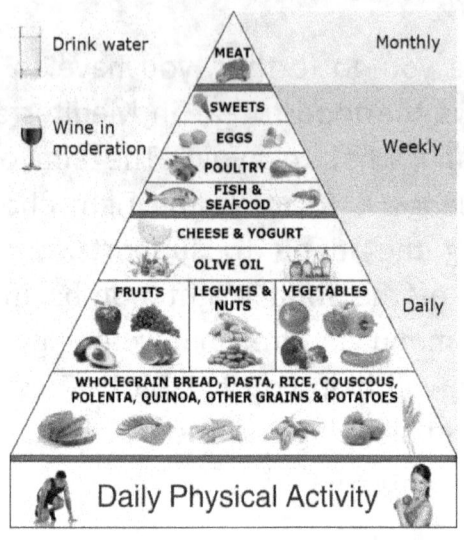

Meal Plan:
Start from day 3, you are recommended to choose the menu based on the Mediterranean food pyramid. Pick four kinds of food in the pyramid that you like. Do not care about line levels, but choose only the listed food.

Breakfast	Lunch	Dinner	Snack
Spinach and Mushroom	Fruit Salads and	Roasted Pork and Mashed	Kale Chips

Omelets	Avocado Juice	Potato

Day 4

Pro Diet Tips:
Eat plenty of vegetables! There is no success diet without vegetables, as they are source of many nutrients, including potassium, fiber, folic acid, vitamins A, E, and C, which are good for your body. Broccoli, spinach, cauliflower, and many other vegetables contain benefits and make them a super food. Again, because of their super benefits, you have to put them as priority in your daily menu.

Meal Plan:
Lucky you, there are so many choices of vegetables that offer good taste. With little help from herbs and spices, vegetables can taste as good as potato chips in your hands.

Breakfast	Lunch	Dinner	Snack
Roasted Pumpkin and	Lettuce and Bacon	Asparagus Soup*	Spinach Chips

| Steamed Cassava | Taco | and Garlic Bread | |

*The recipe is available in the last chapter of the book.

Day 5

Pro Diet Tips:

One kind of food that is recommended in Mediterranean diet is grains. Barley, buckwheat, bulgur, faro, millet, oats, polenta, rice, breads, couscous, and pastas are the examples of common whole grains in Mediterranean area, which are good to consume. In order to make the maximum nutrients in grains, you must have grains in minimal-processed form because refining and processing them in long processes will remove the valuable vitamins, minerals, and fiber.

Meal Plan:

As grains are low fat, low cholesterol, and high carbohydrates, you are suggested to have grain in moderate portion every day. It will be best if you combine with vegetables so that they can make a good cooperation in giving you energy for the whole day. However, in Mediterranean regions, people prefer eating bread plainly or by dipping it in olive oil to having them with butter or margarine, which contains of saturated fats.

Breakfast	Lunch	Dinner	Snack
Peanut Pancake with Maple Syrup*	Chicken Cordon Bleu with Mashed Potato	Roasted Chicken and Lettuce Cucumber Salads	Frozen Banana

*The recipe is available in the last chapter of the book.

Day 6

Pro Diet Tips:

Abalone, clams, cockles, crab, eel, flounder, lobster, mackerel, mussels, octopus, oyster, salmon, sardines, sea bass, shrimps, squid, tilapia, tuna, whelk, and yellowtail are common seafood in Mediterranean diet. Fish and shellfish are the source of animal proteins and they contain Omega 3, which are good for your brain and heart.

Meal Plan:

In order to get enough animal protein during your diet, it is best to have seafood twice a week. Though it is not common to fry fish in Mediterranean, you may fry them as long as you choose healthy oil. Make sure that you have already drained the oil completely before eating the fish and other seafood.

Breakfast	Lunch	Dinner	Snack
Choco Peanut Waffle*	Steamed Vegetables with Peanut Sauce	Smoked Salmon Salad with Carrot and Beans	2 Bites of Brownies

*The recipe is available in the last chapter of the book.

Day 7

Pro Diet Tips:

Another important product that is good according to Mediterranean diet is dairy. Dairy is rich in calcium; which is good for your bones. Besides, it also contains high content of vitamin A, vitamin B12, and protein. Research shows that having dairy product may make you satiated longer so that you will eat less overall. However, it is also known that though full-cream milk is rich in calcium, it is also high in saturated fat. Regarding to that fact, you are recommended to choose semi skimmed milk, low fat yoghurts, and lower fat cheese.

Meal Plan:

Cottage cheese, mozzarella, and feta are some of the low saturated cheese. Consume one of them twice a week is good in applying Mediterranean diet. Beside those kinds of cheese, you can also have milk, yoghurt, butter, or cream to support your need of dairy product.

Breakfast	Lunch	Dinner	Snack
A Glass of Fresh Milk and a Slice of Garlic Bread	Sautéed Bok Choi and Fried Tofu	Homemade Pizza with Mozzarella	Steamed Corn and Cheese

Day 8

Pro Diet Tips:

Another food that is recommended to consume is fruit. There is a wide range of delicious fruits you can have. From fresh orange, apple, banana, melon or fig, to pomegranate, strawberry, grape, and peaches. Whole fresh fruit is available in the Mediterranean. As fruits have lots of benefit, the Mediterranean diet advises you to have fruits every day.

Meal Plan:

Instead of having ice cream, cookies, or mini cake, fruit is much better for dessert. Encourage your family to consume fruit everyday to get the whole benefits. You can eat it rights way, make puree, or juice.

The main thing you have to know is that: do not put additional sugar in the fruit, as it will add unnecessary calories that may ruin your diet. Start from day 8, please put fruit in your daily menu. Have a variety of fruit to avoid you feeling bored. Besides that, you have to know that any kinds of fruit drink are not a choice in Mediterranean diet.

Breakfast	Lunch	Dinner	Snack
Blueberry Muffin	Ebi Furai and Avocado Sushi	Chicken Pineapple Skewers and Roasted Eggplant	Banana Cookies Smoothie

Day 9

Pro Diet Tips:

Nuts and seeds also take an important role in Mediterranean diet. The high content of protein, fiber, vitamin, and mineral may help you to control your weight. As they have a high content of saturated fat, nuts and seed also protect you against heart disease, diabetes, and bad cholesterol. Almond, chestnut, walnut, and cashew are the example of nuts recommended in Mediterranean diet, while pumpkin, sunflower, sesame, and poppy are seeds that offer you their good nutrients.

Meal Plan:

A handful of unsalted nuts is enough for your snack. Beside that, you can also add an amount of sesame or sunflower seeds to a bowl of vegetable salads. It will give you better taste and sensation.

Breakfast	Lunch	Dinner	Snack
Carrot Tomato Omelets*	Shrimps Roll and Brown Rice	Sautéed Broccoli and Grilled Tuna in Barbeque Sauce	A Handful of Roasted Cashew

*The recipe is available in the last chapter of the book.

Day 10

Pro Diet Tips:

Red meat is allowed as well in Mediterranean diet. Because red meat contains saturated fat that can increase the cardiovascular diseases and cholesterol, the Mediterranean diet put this kind of food on the top of the pyramid, which means that red meat may be consumed less often. In order to get the maximum benefits with the lowest risk of beef, lamb, and pork, pick the lean cuts as they contain less fat.

Meal Plan:

If you want to consume red meat, it is recommended to have organic or grass-fed meat. Besides the organic meat contains less fat, it also hormones free and safe to be consume. Have a little amount of red meat in your menu to give better taste for your food.

Breakfast	Lunch	Dinner	Snack
A Glass of Fresh Milk and	Mixed Vegetables Salads	Lamb Chopped with	Frozen Banana

| Waffle with Raw Honey | with Olive Dressing* | Mushroom Sauce and Steamed Vegetables |

*The recipe is available in the last chapter of the book.

Day 11

Pro Diet Tips:
Chicken, turkey, and other poultry or often called as white meat are also good food in Mediterranean diet. For the best result, you are recommended to have lean white meat without skin, as it is high in protein, vitamin B12, and minerals and less saturated fat than red meat. However, chicken burger, turkey fast food, and other junk food are generally high in saturated animal fat and do not count as lean white meat.

Meal Plan:
After 10 days of starting Mediterranean diet, hopefully you can have better menu

to satisfy your craving. You can start to make a week meal plan for you and your family so that the whole family will get the good advantages of applying Mediterranean diet as well.

Breakfast	Lunch	Dinner	Snack
Cheese Tomato Sandwich	Chicken Teriyaki* and Brown Rice	Vegetables Salad and Roasted Turkey	Fish and Chips

*The recipe is available in the last chapter of the book.

Day 12

Pro Diet Tips:
Beside meat, dairy, and fish, another alternative for this diet is egg. Duck, chicken, and quail eggs are all common to traditional Mediterranean diet. Furthermore, the eggs can be a substitute for those who do not want to consume meat and fish. As good as meat, eggs are also rich in high quality protein. However, since eggs contain of animal fat, it is

recommended to consume less often so you will get the maximum result without having the bad effect for consuming too many eggs.

Meal Plan:

There are lots of ways of eating eggs that you can try. The eggs can be boiled, fried with good oil, make it scrambled and omelet, and many more. To reach the best benefit of eggs and to give more tasty meal, you can add any kinds of vegetables so that you can get both protein and vitamin.

Breakfast	Lunch	Dinner	Snack
Onion and Cherry Tomato Scrambled Egg	Chicken Curry Burritos	Lentil soup and Crab in Oyster Sauce	Piece of Fruits

Day 13

Pro Diet Tips:

It can be denied that it is difficult to leave oil at all because most of food is cooked using oil. However, we have to be wise in choosing the best oil to consume, which is still friendly to Mediterranean diet. Until now, extra virgin olive oil is still the best choice for Mediterranean diet that is rich in unsaturated fats and important micronutrients. Olive oil is on the second place and can be used for cooking, baking, and as dressing for salads. Besides the two kinds of oil above, there are some good oils that you can use, such as: canola oil, safflower oil, sesame oil, and tahini.

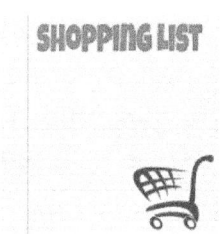

Meal Plan:
As you have already known the kinds of food that are good to support the Mediterranean diet, on day 13 you can start to make a shopping list so that you

only bring health and right ingredients to your home.

Breakfast	Lunch	Dinner	Snack
A Slice of Toast with Pineapple Jam	Vegetables Salads with Olive Dressing	Roasted Chicken with Raw Honey and Beans	Fruit Bars

Day 14

Pro Diet Tips: Though sweets are also in the Mediterranean diet pyramid, they are put on the top of the pyramid. The purpose of this arrangement is to show that sweets are prohibited to consume less. As many products of sweet are high in sugar, saturated fats, and calories, Mediterranean diet only permits you to consume sweet once a month as a celebration or treat. It is done for sweet foods damage teeth; increase heart diseases, diabetes, and obesity.

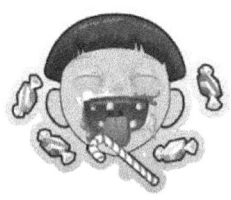

Meal Plan:

After having two weeks of Mediterranean diet without breaking the rules, you will feel that your body is stronger and energetic. This health condition will be the best weapon for you to do all your daily activities perfectly.

Breakfast	Lunch	Dinner	Snack
Cheese Banana Pancake	Sautéed Broccoli with Meat Balls	Chicken and Corn Soup and Potato Wedges	Yogurt and Cranberries

Day 15

Pro Diet Tips:
Being put in the bottom of Mediterranean diet pyramid, it is shown that herbs and spices are remarkably healthy and good to be consumed daily. The Mediterranean added herbs and spices into their cuisines to get tempting aromas and scrumptious flavors. Besides, by adding herbs and spices, you can reduce the amount of salt into your meal. Basil, bay leaf, sage, rosemary, savory, garlic, fennel, cumin, sage, thyme, and cloves are the examples of herb and spices. Nevertheless, only use fresh herbs and spices to give different touch to your meal.

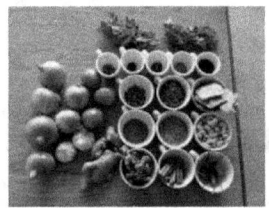

Meal Plan:
Now, you have already in the middle of first step of Mediterranean diet. Sometimes it is difficult to follow the rule and avoid the prohibited food, which

usually is more tempting. However, if you have passed this half step, it will be easier for you to continue. It is shown that your body has adjusted the Mediterranean diet so it will be easier for you to continue.

Breakfast	Lunch	Dinner	Snack
Garlic Bread with Honey and Raisin	Spaghetti Bolognese	Asian Beef Curry* and Steamed Vegetables	Cassava Chips

*The recipe is available in the last chapter of the book.

Day 16

Pro Diet Tips:

It is fascinating to know that wine is good and also allowed in Mediterranean diet. Wine, which is made from grape skins and seeds, contains powerful antioxidant and useful as an anti aging. Men are advised to have two glass of wine per day to help them prevent strokes while having one glass of wine every day is enough for woman.

Meal Plan:

From day 16 you have to try to make all family dishes especially dinner. Cook your dinner and eat it with your family on the dining table. After dinner, you can have an intimate conversation with the beloved ones while enjoying wine in your portion. If you refuse to have wine, you can drink a glass of fresh grape juice without sugar

Breakfast	Lunch	Dinner	Snack
Bacon and Cheese Scrambled Egg*	Steamed Vegetables and Roasted Shrimps	Beef Spicy Burritos	Grape Juice

*The recipe is available in the last chapter of the book.

Day 17

Pro Diet Tips:

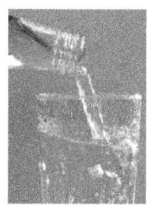

Similar to what every diet does, Mediterranean diet advises you to drink at least 8 glasses of water to keep you hydrated. Have enough water weather you are on diet or not, is good for the body metabolism as water is a natural detox and can help you to burn more calories in your body.

Meal Plan:

Drink a glass of water before eating is good, as it will help you to control your meal portion. Day by day you have to increase the amount of water you can drink and reduce the consumption of coffee and soda.

Breakfast	Lunch	Dinner	Snack
Carrot Muffins	Spicy Sandwich Tofu and Fruit	Asparagus Soup and Chicken	A Handful of Grapes

Salads	Meatballs

Day 18

Pro Diet Tips:

There is no healthy lifestyle without exercising. In order to get the perfect results of Mediterranean diet, you have to combine the good eating habits with regular exercises. Not only the exercise helps you to burn excess calories and fat, but it also helps you to give a better body shape. Men will be more gallant while the women will be sexier. Surely, you will be glad to have this benefit of having a combination between healthy diet and exercises.

Meal Plan:

To start the high quality exercise, you have to take at least 30 minutes of daily exercise. It will be hard in the beginning, but once you feel the effects, you will enjoy of having them daily. You can start with jogging or cycling around your home every morning. If you are too busy to do that, try to do simple move during your daily activities. Instead of using elevator, take stairs to move to different floors.

Breakfast	Lunch	Dinner	Snack
Roasted Sausage and Potato Wedges	Tomato and Tuna Taco	Roasted Beef in Peanut Sauce with Sautéed Broccoli	A Handful of Roasted Cashew

Day 19

Pro Diet Tips:

Having 8 hours of sleeping is important for your Mediterranean diet. While you are sleeping your body is working to burn your fat and reduce weight. On the other side, if you are lack of sleep, you will only get 50 % of fat burning. Thus, it is really recommended for you to get enough sleep, reduce the stress level, and have a double chance to slimming down your body.

Meal Plan:

As traditional herbs, nutmeg is a good example to help you to get good quality of sleeping. A teaspoon of nutmeg in your dinner will help you to sleep tight and have a sweet dream. The other thing you should do during the relaxation is, turn your smart phone off and put it far away from you so you can have completely time to rest. Sleeping with dim light or no light at all is also recommended to assure that your body is totally relaxed.

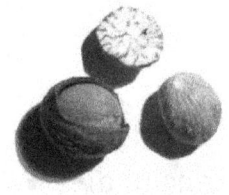

Breakfast	Lunch	Dinner	Snack
Roasted Tomato with Mozzarella Cheese	Roasted Salmon with Broccoli Popcorn	Chicken Carrot Soup with Nutmeg	Steamed Carrot with Mayonnaise

		Powder and Fried Tempeh

Day 20

Pro Diet Tips:

Consuming food from the Mediterranean diet is a very good and discipline action. However, every single person has various needs of calories. It depends on the body size and activities. So, if you want to achieve the goal of having ideal weight, you have to concern on the amount of the food you take. If you consume too many calories than you need, it will be a surplus of energy for your body and will be stored as fat.

Meal Plan:

From day 20, try to cook the food you are going to eat. Besides, you can make an appropriate portion, you will also avoid from having bad substances like MSG. No wonder that almost all restaurants add

MSG to their food to serve better and tempted tastes.

Breakfast	Lunch	Dinner	Snack
Almond Waffle and Chocolate Sauce	Chicken Curry Kebab with Fresh Lettuce	Roasted Pumpkin and Chicken Strips	Bacon Rissoles

Day 21

Pro Diet Tips:

Do your diet happily. Actually, any kinds of diet will achieve their best result if the applicants are enjoying every step of the dieting method. If it possible, does the diet with some friends or family so you can support each other. Besides, you can have a "positive competition" between you and your partner so everybody will be eager to reach the highest goal of the diet.

Meal Plan:

Cook your lunch at double portions and share it with your colleagues at the office. Having a healthy lunch from home with partner may avoid you from being tempted for less healthy meal from the cafeteria.

Breakfast	Lunch	Dinner	Snack
Fruit Salads	Butternut Squash Casserole	Mac and Cheese	Chicken Popcorn

Day 22

Pro Diet Tips:

Take a world tour in your kitchen. Make friend with all kitchen equipment's that will be your best partners in cooking healthy food for your diet. Keep your pantry clean and as cozy as you can so you will enjoy spending your time to cook there. Besides, a clean and neat kitchen also serves quality food as it keeps the high quality ingredients from cockroach, mice, or other yucky things coming from dirty kitchen.

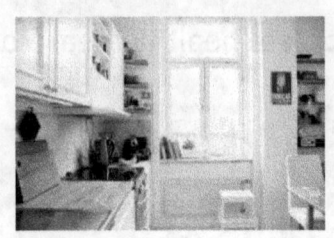

Meal Plan:

Fill your refrigerator with the food that is available in the Mediterranean pyramid. If you have busy days, you can store many fresh ingredients in your refrigerator and take it in several minutes before cooking. From now on, you have to avoid of having canned food because they are not preservative free and will give bad effect for you.

Breakfast	Lunch	Dinner	Snack
Green Beans Frittata	Fried Noodles with Ebi Furai	Spinach Salmon Roll and Brown	Strawberry Smoothies

| | | Rice | |

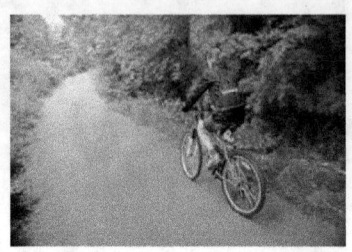

Day 23

Pro Diet Tips:

Embrace sunshine and have fun!! Outside activities are always good for those who want to be healthier. You may be afraid of the ultraviolet, but as long as you have the outside activities in the morning, you will not be burnt by its side effects. Even, the morning sun will help your body to process vitamin D, and it will keep you away from horrible osteoporosis.

Meal Plan:

At least once a week, try to be vegetarian. Consume vegetables as they can be cooked in many different ways. Don't worry, there are lots of recipes that you can find and try. Having vegetable for the day, without meat at all, will give a good stomach condition in the next morning.

Breakfast	Lunch	Dinner	Snack
Brownies and Fresh Cherry	Mushroom Risotto	Italian Beef Steak and Steamed Carrot	Potato Chips

Day 24

Pro Diet Tips:

If you have already had kids, encourage your kids to have this Mediterranean eating habits from the beginning so they will have a healthy life style when they grow up. Be a role model for your kids so that they will learn how important the health it is from you.

Meal Plan:

Be patient to your kids in teaching them to consume good and healthy food. Set your mind that kids are dynamic person. It is usual to understand that they will change their habits relatively easier than you. So, you have to make various meals plan and decorate it according your capability to increase their appetite.

Breakfast	Lunch	Dinner	Snack
Roasted Potato with Cheese Sauce and Celery	Caesar Salad	Fresh Crab Spaghetti	A Handful of Peanut

Day 25

Pro Diet Tips:

Mediterranean diet is not as hard as another diet. It permits you to have anything you want, from healthy fruits and vegetables to high fat red meat and sweet. However, you have to pay attention a lot on how you consume them, the portion size, and the balance of food intake.

Meal Plan:

After 24 days of Mediterranean diet, you

will be familiar to the allowed food and be able to create weekly plan menu easily.

Breakfast	Lunch	Dinner	Snack
Fresh Orange and Pear	Steamed Vegetables with Peanut Sauce	American Pie and Steamed Vegetables	A Bowl of Cubed Mango

Day 26

Pro Diet Tips:
Mediterranean diet is not about the physical thing. Further more, having Mediterranean diet is like having a journey that teaches you about reaching goal, adjust strategy and being patience. Collaborate Mediterranean diet with self-development will result a good combination both physically and mentally.

Meal Plan:
Be creative in creating menu and enjoy having the Mediterranean diet as your lifestyle. Try to mix a little amount of meat with a bunch of vegetables to get a better

taste of food but still healthy enough to be consumed.

Breakfast	Lunch	Dinner	Snack
Peanut Pancake	Steamed Kale and Fish Meatball	Chicken Cheese Casserole	Frozen Banana

Day 27

Pro Diet Tips:

As a social human being, there is always a chance to hang out with some friends. Besides, you will be invited to a party, gathering, or other occasional meeting. Although you are in Mediterranean diet, you still can be a part of the cheerfulness. Instead of eating nothing, you can try to pick the healthiest menu on the table. But if you fail to find it, you may enjoy the food served but you have to pay attention to the portion.

Meal Plan:

When you are in the restaurant, ask the server for the dieting menu in the restaurant. If it is possible, request them to serve organic menu without MSG and high content of salt.

Breakfast	Lunch	Dinner	Snack
Banana Raisin Waffle	Mac and Cheese	Beef Steak with Mashed Potato and Fresh Lettuce	Potato Chips

Day 28

Pro Diet Tips:

After four weeks of Mediterranean diet, get back to the first goal of having this diet. If you feel that this Mediterranean diet hasn't given your desire result yet, do not temp to quit. Maybe there is something that you did not do it correctly. Check out what is not working on you, adjust your strategy, and achieve your best goal.

Meal Plan:

As Mediterranean diet is not a kind of

fads, try to stay on the path and choose healthy menu for your healthier lifestyle.

Breakfast	Lunch	Dinner	Snack
Sausage and Green Beans Omelets	Butternut Squash and Mushroom Risotto	Beef Tomato Lasagna	Steam Kale and Money Bag

Day 29

Pro Diet Tips:

Again, you can understand that the main principles of Mediterranean diet are eating fruits and vegetables every day, have any kinds of seafood several times a week, and having a smaller portion of beef, poultry and grain. Beans and lentils can be consumed more often. Instead of using butter and lard, use the healthy fats like olive oil.

Meal Plan:

In the forth week of applying the Mediterranean diet, you will completely understand on how to manage your body weight and metabolism. Adjust your menu according to the Mediterranean pyramid.

Nevertheless, if you want to cheat, do it right for a day and then get back to the principles of Mediterranean diet the day after.

Breakfast	Lunch	Dinner	Snack
A Slice of Toast with Blueberry Jam	Tofu Meatball and Sautéed Vegetables	Asparagus Soup, Fish and Chips, and Potato Wedges	A Handful of Roasted Cashew

Day 30

Pro Diet Tips:

Now, you have been in Mediterranean diet for a month. Obviously, every dieting method has its own difficulties, and maybe you have thought that Mediterranean diet was hard to be applied. However, today you have found that Mediterranean diet is not as complicated as the theory if you enjoy them naturally and eagerly.

Meal Plan:

To satisfy your appetite, cook some meal

that includes your favorite food, as long as it is Mediterranean friendly. As there are many kinds of ingredients that are suggested in Mediterranean diet, you can make various serving for your lunch and dinner.

Breakfast	Lunch	Dinner	Snack
Carrot Muffins	Fruit Salads	Roasted Pork with Honey Sauce	Spinach Chips

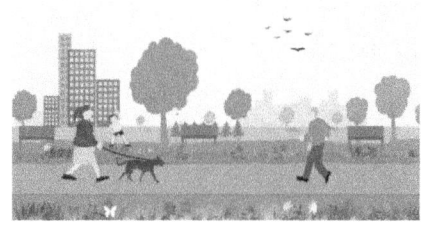

Day 31

Pro Diet Tips:
Congratulations for having the first month program of Mediterranean diet!! It is clear that you are now in a healthier lifestyle. All the programs and meal plans help you to maintain your body appearance and metabolism to reach better health. Stay on the Mediterranean, follow the pyramid and have a wonderful life, healthy people!!

Meal Plan:
Continue to arrange your menu according to the Mediterranean pyramid. Be thankful for the life given and enjoy it as a perfect blessing from above.

Breakfast	Lunch	Dinner	Snack
A Slice of Toast with Pineapple Jam	Vegetable Salads with Toss of olive Dressing	Spinach Chicken Casserole	Piece of Fruits

Mediterranean Diet Recipes

Fortunately, this diet book provides many recipes that may help you to prepare healthy food for your beloved ones. The recipes in this book are selectively chosen for those who pay attention a lot in having good health. So, what are you waiting for? Try and enjoy the recipes below, and be healthy!!

Roasted Salmon with Black Pepper Sauce

Ingredients:
2 salmon fillets
1 tablespoon honey
½ tablespoon mustard
½ teaspoon lemon juice

1 teaspoon black pepper

Instructions:

Drizzle salmon with lemon juice and sat aside for half an hour.

Place all remaining ingredients in a small bowl, and stir together until well combined.

Place the salmon fillets on the baking sheet and drizzle with the black pepper sauce.

Bake for about 10 minutes or until the salmon is enough cooked.

Serve immediately.

Chicken Cheese in Roll

Ingredients:

2 chicken breasts
4 tablespoons shredded cheddar cheese
2 tablespoons softened cream cheese
1 tablespoon olive oil
2 tablespoons chutney

Instructions:

Place the chicken on the flat surface.

Combine the shredded cheddar cheese and cream cheese, than spread evenly over the chicken.
Roll the chicken and secure with a toothpick.
Combine the olive oil and chutney then grease onto the chicken roll.
Bake the chicken at 350 °F for approximately 30 minutes.
Serve right away.

Mixed Vegetables Salads with Olive Dressing

Ingredients:
1 cup cubed potatoes
½ cup cubed carrot
1 tablespoon chopped parsley
½ cup cubed apple
½ cup cubed cucumber
¼ cup green peas
2 tablespoons olive oil
Instructions:

Boil carrots and potatoes, then drain them and place into a medium bowl with lid.

Add in all remaining ingredients into the bowl, and then toss them together.

Refrigerate the salads for about 20 minutes.

Transfer the salads to a serving dish.

Serve immediately.

Asparagus Soup

Ingredients:
1 cup chopped asparagus
1 tablespoon chopped shallot
1 tablespoon crushed garlic
1 cup chopped spinach
1 tablespoon olive oil
2 cups chicken broth

Instructions:
Preheat the olive oil in a saucepan.

Add the asparagus into the saucepan and fry until soften, set aside.

Add in the shallots and garlic, and then cook for about 5 minutes until smooth.

Add in spinach, stir together until wilted.

Pour the broth into the saucepan and cook until boiled.
Let the soup cool for about 1 minutes, then blitz using a hand blender.
Serve right away.

Peanut Pancake with Maple Syrup

Ingredients:
½ cup fresh milk
½ cup granulated sugar
4 tablespoons peanut butter
½ teaspoon vanilla extract
½ cup maple syrup

Instructions:
Place all ingredients except the maple syrup into a bowl.
Stir them together until incorporated.
Preheat a saucepan, and then pour the pancake batter into the saucepan evenly.
Cook pancake for about 3 minutes.
Remove from heat and transfer to a plate.
Drizzle maple syrup over the pancake.
Enjoy right away.

Choco Peanut Waffle

Ingredients:
1 cup all-purpose flour
2 teaspoons baking powder
4 tablespoons crunchy peanut butter
1 tablespoon cocoa powder
1 tablespoon sugar
1 egg, lightly beaten
1 cup fresh milk
2 tablespoons olive oil
Cooking spray

Instructions:
Place all ingredients in a medium bowl.
Stir gradually all ingredients until incorporated.
Preheat the waffle iron and spray with cooking spray.
Once the waffle iron is preheated, pour the batter into the waffle iron.
Cook for about 3 minutes, serve warm.

Carrot Tomato Omelets

Ingredients:
4 eggs, lightly beaten
½ cup grated carrot
½ cup diced tomato
¼ teaspoon black pepper
¼ teaspoon salt

Instructions:
Combine all ingredients in a medium bowl and stir until incorporated.
Preheat a pan and spray with cooking spray, wait until the pan is hot.
Pour the omelets batter into the pan and cook for approximately 15 minutes.
Serve immediately.

Chicken Teriyaki

Ingredients:
1 tablespoons sake
2 tablespoons mirin
2 tablespoons soya sauce
1 tablespoon brown sugar
1 teaspoon gingerroot powder
1 teaspoon sesame oil

1 cup chicken fillet

½ teaspoon peanut oil

Instructions:

Marinate chicken with sake, mirin, soy sauce, sugar, ginger, and sesame oil for 15 minutes.

Heat the peanut oil in a skillet over medium heat.

Transfer the marinated chicken into the skillet, the sauté it until golden brown.

Continue to cook for about 5 minutes, or until the chicken is totally cooked.

Once it is done, remove the chicken teriyaki onto a serving dish.

Best to serve with warm Japanese rice.

Asian Beef Curry

Ingredients:

300 grams beef, cut into bite size pieces

3 lemon grass, bruised and cut

100 ml tamarind water

½ teaspoon sugar

3 vegetable oil

2 bay leaves

1500 ml water
200 ml coconut milk
½ handful scallions, finely chopped
½ celery leaves, finely chopped
SPICES
5 cloves garlic
4 grains candlenut
2 teaspoons pepper powder
1 cm fresh turmeric
a pinch of salt
GARNISH:
1 tablespoon fried onion
2 kaffir lime, cut into quarters

Instructions :

In a food processor, blend all the spices ingredients.

Heat vegetable oil in a soup pot and stir fry spice paste, bay leaves and lemon grass until fragrant, about 2-3 minutes.

Add the beef into the pot, mix well until the beef is coated with the spices. Add in sugar and tamarind water then cook until the color starts to change.

Pour the water and bring to a boil. Reduce the heat, cover and simmer for about 1

hour, or until the meat is fully cooked and tender.
Pour the coconut milk, stir then bring to a boil again.
Once it boils, immediately turn of the heat, add the scallions and celery leaves.
Once it is done, transfer to a bowl and garnish with fried onion.
Serve immediately with steamed white rice and a squeeze of kaffir lime juice.

Bacon and Cheese Scrambled Egg

Ingredients:
½ cup chopped bacon
2 large eggs, lightly beaten
1 tablespoon fresh milk
¼ cup grated cheese
¼ cup chopped onion
¼ teaspoon pepper
¼ teaspoon salt
1 teaspoon olive oil
Instructions:
Sauté the bacon on a saucepan until crispy, and then set aside.

Combine all ingredients except olive oil in a bowl, and then stir gradually until incorporated.

Preheat olive oil in a saucepan, and then pour the eggs batter into the saucepan.

Keep tossing the batter with a spatula to make it scrambled.

Once it is cooked, remove to the serving dish.

Enjoy immediately.

Conclusion

Congratulation on your determination to choose Mediterranean diet. The complete information presents in this book can absolutely give you the right guidance in having Mediterranean diet. In all seriousness, this book is made to show you the simplest way to have a healthier way of eating. It is more about how to appreciate life by having a healthy lifestyle and furthermore, to have a beautiful life. As dieting method is a process, do not stop if you haven't reached your target in loosing weight yet. Healthy body and good metabolism will be the first goal of having a good lifestyle, and loosing weight is like an extra bonus. Stay on the path of Mediterranean diet, do the good eating habit and attain longer healthy life.

Thank you and good luck.

Part 2

Breakfast Recipes

Cookies With Peanut Butter

Ingredients

- 1 large egg
- Peanut butter (¾ cup), chunky
- Baking mix (½ cup)
- Almond flour (½ cup)
- Salt (¼ tsp)
- Baking soda (1 tsp)
- Butter (½ cup), softened
- Splenda sugar substitute (½ cup)
- Vital wheat gluten (2 tsp)
- Oat flour (½ cup)
- Brown sugar twin (½ cup)

Direction

Blend egg along with sweetener and butter until smooth.

Put in peanut butter and mix well.

Afterward, add dry ingredients and mix well.

Now make balls from the mixture and press with spoon.

Baking in the preheated oven for about 15 minutes at 375 degrees Fahrenheit until browned.

Spinach Salad-Greek Version

Ingredients

- Olive oil (¼ cup)
- 1 garlic clove, minced
- Cheese (8 ounces), crumbled
- ½ red onion, sliced thinly
- Baby spinach (1 package), steamed, washed and drained
- Walnut (¼ cup), coarsely chopped
- Roasted red pepper (2 ounces), drained, cut into strips and patted
- Red vinegar (3 tbsp)

Direction

Mix garlic and vinegar in a large mixing bowl.

Add oil and whisk constantly to become homogenous and steady.

Put in onion and spinach and mix well until coated.

Now add pepper strips and cheese and then potion the mixture into the plate.

Splash with walnuts and then serve.

Special Coleslaw

Ingredients

- Dry mustard (1 tsp)
- Sugar (¼ cup)
- Vegetable (¼ cup)
- 1 head of cabbage, shredded thinly
- Salt (1 tsp)
- Hot sauce (½ tsp)
- White vinegar (½ cup)

Direction

Whisk all the ingredients together and then pour into a cabbage.

Toss them well and chill before serving.

Paleo Pudding

Ingredients

- Frozen raspberry (¼ cup)
- Honey (1 tbsp)
- Unsweetened almond milk (1 cup)
- Protein powder (1 scoop)
- Chia seeds (3 tbsp)

Direction

Combine protein powder, chocolate and almond milk together and stir well.

Mix in chia seeds and then let it stand for about 5 minutes.

Stir again and then reserve for 5 minutes more.

Now chill in the refrigerator for about 30 minutes.

Top with raspberries while serving.

Spinach Omelet

Ingredients

- Cooking spray
- Garlic (optional)
- Purple onion (1 tbsp)
- Basil (1 pinch)
- 1 plum tomato
- 1 handful of shredded spinach
- 1 egg yolk
- Almond milk (2 tbsp)
- 4-5 egg whites

Direction

Beat yolk, almond milk and egg whites together.

Chop vegetables.

Spray a saucepan with oil and sauté the vegetables in it until tender.

Set the veggies aside.

Now add egg mixture to the center of the pan and cook until the eggs are set.

Add veggies over the top.

Also top with some fruits if desired and then serve.

Hot Cereal

Ingredients

- Heavy cream (2 tbsp)
- A dash of cinnamon
- Sweetener according to taste
- 1 pinch salt
- Boiling water (1/3 cup)
- Shredded coconut meat (1 ½ tbsp)
- Flax seed meal (1 tbsp)
- Ground pecans (1 ½ tbsp)

Direction

Combine coconut, pecans and flax seed meals together in a bowl, add salt and then stir well.

Now add boiling water and mix well so that water incorporates evenly with the mixture.

Reserve for few minutes and then add cream and sweetener before serving.

Fat Scramble

Ingredients

- Small beef cubes (1 tbsp)
- Cheddar cheese (1/8 cup)
- Melted butter (2 tsp)
- Heavy cream (2 tsp)
- 1 egg
- Olive oil (1 tbsp)

Direction

Take a saucepan and spray with olive oil.

Beat cream, eggs, pepper, salt and butter together.

Now put the pan over the stove on medium high heat and add egg mixture.

Mix until the eggs are done using spatula.

Put in cheese and beef and mix well until the eggs are done and the cheese has melted.

Tea Special

Ingredients

- Splenda sugar substitute (2 packets)
- Ground cloves (1 pinch)
- Coriander (1 pinch)
- Heavy cream (4 ounces)
- Ground cinnamon (1 pinch)
- Ground ginger (1 pinch)
- Cold tea (12 ounces)

Direction

Combine all the ingredients and mix well. Transfer into a cup and serve cold.

Burrito Breakfast Style

Ingredients

- Chili powder (1 tbsp)
- Vegetable oil (1 tbsp)
- 2 whole wheat tortillas
- 4 pieces of eggs
- 1 red chili pepper
- Red bell pepper (1 piece)

- Spring onion (2 pieces)

Direction

Beat eggs with cayenne and salt together.

Heat oil in a pan and cook wheat tortillas on each side in it.

Cover the tortillas with aluminum foil to keep them warm.

Add vegetable oil to the pan and sauté spring onion, red bell pepper and red chili pepper in it.

Put in egg mixture and mix for about 2 minutes until cooked.

Now transfer the mixture to the tortillas and roll them up.

Serve and enjoy.

Banana And Cheese

Ingredients
- Ground cinnamon (1 tbsp)
- Half fresh banana
- Cheese (40 gm)

- Whole wheat bread, 1 slice

Direction

Slice banana vertically.

Toast bread slice and spread the cheese over it followed by banana slice.

Splash with ground cinnamon and serve.

Egg And Cheese Sandwich

Ingredients

- Cheddar cheese (30 gm)
- Whole wheat bread, 2 slices
- 1 piece of egg
- Non-fat milk (20 ml)

Direction

Break egg into the plate without breaking its yolk.

Combine with non-fat milk and add salt to it.

Put in the microwave for about 2 minutes until done.

Take the bread slices and toast it.

Put the cooked egg on the bread slice and splash with cheese followed by the other slice of bread over it.

Microwave it again until the cheese is melted, for about 15 minutes and then serve.

Almond, Blueberries And Cheese

Ingredients

- 24 pieces of roasted almonds
- Fresh blueberries (40 gm)
- Cheese (150 gm)

Direction

Take cheese in a bowl and splash with chopped almonds.

Top with blueberries and serve.

Veggie Omelet

Ingredients

- Butter (2 tbsp), softened
- Pepper (2 tbsp)
- 1 medium size fresh onion, whites
- Iodized salt (1 tbsp)
- 6 pieces of eggs
- Red pepper (1 piece)
- Green bell pepper (1 piece)
- Soya milk (40 ml), unsweetened
- Mozzarella cheese (100 gm)

Direction

Minced onion and pepper and keep them aside.

Take a frying pan and melt butter in it.

Put in minced pepper and onion and cook for about 4 minutes.

Scramble eggs, beat it with soya milk and salt and mix well.

Now pour the egg mixture to the pan and cook for about 2 minutes.

Mix vegetables and onion well.

Top with mozzarella cheese, invert the egg and then cook further for about 2 minutes.

Serve and enjoy.

Protein Crepes

Ingredients

- Baking soda (½ tsp)
- 3 egg whites
- Makes 4 crepes
- Ground flaxseed (2 tbsp)
- Almond milk
- Unsweetened (¼ cup)
- 2 large eggs
- Coconut flour (¼ cup)

Direction

Take a food processor; combine all the ingredients in it and process.

Now take a pan spray with cooking oil and then add the above mixture in a circular shape.

Cook until the bubble comes out.

Flip and cook on the other side and serve when cool.

Broccoli Cheese Soup

Ingredients

- Cheddar cheese (1 cup)
- Pepper to taste
- Salt (1 tsp)
- Heavy whipping cream (¼ cup)
- Half cup of chicken broth
- Softened cream cheese (4 ounces)
- Water (2 cups)
- Broccoli florets (2 cups)

Direction

Steam broccoli floret until done.

Take a blender and add half cup of water, half cup of broccoli, heavy cream and cream cheese.

Blend until smooth.

Now shift the mixture to the frying pan and add the remaining water, broccoli and chicken broth.

Mix well and simmer on low heat.

Put in cheddar cheese and mix until the cheese is absorbed by the mixture.

Flavor it with pepper before serving.

Lime Cheese Cake

Ingredients

- 3 whole eggs
- Artificial sweetener equal to 12 tsp sugar
- True lime (6 packets)
- Heavy whipping cream (½ cup)
- Softened cream cheese (8 ounces)

Direction

Mix cream cheese and heavy cream in an electric mixture until smooth.

Add rest of the ingredients and blend well.

Use ramekin for batter, lined and greased and add to the cookie sheet.

Bake at 350 Degrees Fahrenheit for about half hour and then place on the rack to cool.

After that put it in the refrigerator and serve once it is cooled.

Asian Noodles

Ingredients

- 1 scallion
- 1 garlic cloves
- Soy sauce (1 tsp)
- Grated ginger root (½ tsp)
- Chicken broth (1 tbsp)
- Liquid stevia (1 drop)
- Dark sesame oil (½ tsp)
- Coconut oil (1 tbsp)
- Natural peanut butter (1 tbsp)
- Traditional shirataki noodles (1 packet)

Direction

Split the noodles, rinse and then drain water.

Take a bowl, put in noodles and nuke for about few minutes. Then drain.

Nuke for further 2 minutes.

Separate noodles by using fork and then add rest of the ingredients.

Mix well until form a sauce.

Top with scallion before serving.

Scrambled Eggs

Ingredients

- Ground pepper (1 pinch)
- Salt (1 pinch)
- 3 large eggs
- Unsalted butter (1 tbsp)

Direction

Take a saucepan and melt butter in it.

Beat eggs and add to the saucepan.

Cook for about 2 minutes until the watery part run out.

Flavor it with pepper and salt.

Lunch Recipes

Lemon Chicken Soup

Ingredients

- Fresh lemon (1 tbsp), squeezed
- Oregano
- Pepper and salt according to taste
- Half small onion, finely minced
- 1 carrot, sliced
- 1 chicken bouillon cube
- 1 egg
- Chicken broth (1 cup)
- Cooked chicken (1 cup), cut into half inch thick pieces

Direction

Combine chicken bouillon, water (1 cup) and chicken broth in a Dutch oven and boil for about 20 minutes until the chicken is tender.

Put in lemon juice and egg over it and splash with salt and pepper.

Add oregano while serving.

Beef Broccoli

Ingredients

- Water (1/8 cup)
- Cornstarch (1 tbsp)
- Soy sauce (1 tbsp)
- Vegetable oil (1 tbsp)
- Water (1 tbsp), divided
- Ginger (¼ tsp), finely grinded
- Garlic powder (1/8 tsp)
- Broccoli florets (1 cup)
- ¼ onion, sliced into wedges
- Round steak (¼ pound), cut into thick strips

Direction

Combine half tsp of cornstarch with water and garlic in a bowl.

Put in beef and mix well.

Now heat half of the oil portion in a saucepan and add coated strips until tender.

Shift the strips to the plate.

Now heat the remaining half oil in a pan and cook broccoli and onions in it for about 4 minutes.

Put in beef strips and mix until browned.

Add cornstarch, soy sauce, water, ginger and sugar and stir for about 2 minutes until completely done.

Serve and enjoy.

Baked Chicken Thighs

Ingredients

- Garlic powder
- 2 chicken thighs
- Soy sauce (2 tbsp)

Direction

Arrange chicken thighs on baking sheet and splash with soy sauce and garlic powder.

Now place in the oven at 350 degrees Fahrenheit for about an hour.

Low Carb Meatballs

Ingredients

- Oregano (¼ tsp)
- Parsley (1/8 cup), chopped
- Pepper and salt to taste
- Onion (1/8 cup), finely chopped
- Breadcrumbs (1/8 cup), made of almond flour
- 1 garlic clove, finely minced
- 1 egg
- Ground beef (½ pound)

Direction

Take a large bowl and combine all the ingredients in it.

Now divide the mixture into three equal portions and then shape each one into round balls.

Put the saucepan over the stove and spray with cooking oil.

Cook meatballs for about 6 minutes on each side until tender.

Serve quickly.

Chicken And Mushrooms

Ingredients

- Garlic powder
- Honey (½ tsp)
- Onion (¼ tbsp), finely minced
- Soy sauce (1 ½ tbsp)
- Green bell pepper (¼ cup), chopped
- Mushroom (1 cup), sliced
- 1 boneless chicken breast

Direction

Preheat the oven to 350 degrees Fahrenheit.

Take baking dish, place the chicken breast over it and Splash with onions.

Mix soy sauce and garlic in a bowl and pour it over chicken.

Cover and cook in the preheated oven for about half hour.

Once cooked, uncover and ad bell pepper and mushroom over the top.

Cover again and bake in the oven until tender.

Allow it to cool for some time and then serve.

Slow Cooker Taco Soup

Ingredients

- Whole kernel corn with liquid (1 can or about 15 ounce)
- Kidney beans with liquid (1 can or 15 ounce)
- Chili beans with liquid (1 can or 16 ounces)
- 1 onion, finely chopped

- Taco seasoning (1 package or 1.25 ounce)
- Green chili pepper (1 can or about 4 ounce)
- Peeled and diced tomatoes (2 cans)
- Water (2 cups)
- Tomato sauce (1 can)
- Ground beef (1 pound)

Direction

Heat oil in a pan and cook ground beef in it until browned. Drain and keep it aside.

Now combine all the ingredients in a slow cooker and mix well.

Minimize the heat and cook for about 8 minutes until ready.

Serve and enjoy the delicious soup.

Slow Cooker Squash

Ingredients

- Processed cheese (¼ pound, cubed)
- Butter (¼ cups, cubed)
- 1 small onion, chopped

- Summer squash (4 pounds, sliced)

Direction

Take water in a pot and put in onion and squash.

Place on the stove and simmer for about 10 minutes until tender.

Drain and then add to the slow cooker.

Make a layer of cheese cubes and butter cubes over the squash mixture and cook on low until butter makes a creamy sauce with cheese. It will take about an hour.

Serve and enjoy the delicious recipe.

Fiesta Bean Dips

Ingredients

- Chunky style salsa (1 jar or 8 ounces)
- Refried beans (1 can or 10 ounces)
- Cheese soup (1 can or 10.75 ounces)
- Sour cream (1 cup)

Direction

Combine cheese soup, refried beans, salsa and sour cream in a pan and cook for about 10 minutes on medium high heat until the mixture is thoroughly warm.

Serve And enjoy.

Rib-Eye And Pepper

Ingredients

- 1 lime, juiced
- Fajita Seasoning (3 tbsp)
- 4 cloves garlic, finely minced
- 1 onion, sliced
- 1 green bell pepper, finely chopped
- 1 red bell pepper, finely chopped
- Beef rib eye steak (4 each of 10 ounce)
- Cooking oil (1 tbsp)

Direction

Take a frying pan and heat oil in it.

Brown steak on both sides in the heated oil and take out.

Put in onion, garlic green and red bell pepper and sauté for about 5 minutes.

Now combine seasoning and steak and put them back to the pan.

Add lime juice to cover the steak and then simmer for about 45 minutes.

Serve when cooked.

Mexican Dip

Ingredients

- Tomatoes and green chilies (1 can)
- 12 Beef tamales, husked and mashed
- Processed cheese (1 loaf)

Direction

Combine all the ingredients in slow cooker and switch the slow cooker to high heat until the cheese is melted.

Reduce the heat and let it keep on the stove to serve warm.

Serve with tortillas.

Roasted Rack Of Lamb, Fennel, Cauliflower And Celery

Ingredients

- Celery (2 cups), sliced
- Cauliflower (2 cups), finely chopped
- Salt according to taste
- Fennel (2 cups), sliced
- Ghee (1 tbsp)
- 1 tbsp of finely chopped fresh thyme, turmeric, rosemary, sage, oregano
- A rack of organic lamb, 1 ½ pound

Direction

Preheat the oven to 350 degrees Fahrenheit.

Mark the lamb and add ghee over it.

Put the vegetables into the pan and then place the lamb over it but make sure that marked fat side is facing up.

Now bake in the preheated oven for about 45 minutes until done.

Now keep the oven on low and bake for further 3 minutes until crisp.

Serve and enjoy.

Sauted Greens And Poached Eggs

Ingredients

- Sliced almond (2 tbsp)
- Kale (2-3 cups)
- Salt according to taste
- 2 eggs, poached
- Unsalted butter (2 tbsp)

Direction

Take frying pan containing water and cook kale in it.

Discard water and then toss it well in butter.

Add salt according to taste and eggs.

Serve with nuts and enjoy.

Salmon Avocado Lunch

Ingredients

- A Hass Avocado
- Cold salmon (4 ounce)
- Salt according to taste

Direction

Slice avocado into 4 inch pieces.

Also slice the salmon into 4 pieces and cover the avocado with the salmon pieces.

Serve and enjoy.

Sweet And Spicy Slow Cooker Chicken

Ingredients

- Raisins (½ cup)
- Tomatoes (1 can or 28 ounces)
- Fresh ginger (3 inch piece, sliced roundly)
- 3 garlic cloves, finely minced
- 1 medium size Yellow onion, cut into half inch wedges along with roots
- Extra – virgin olive oil (1 tbsp)
- Chicken legs (4 pieces)
- Grinded pepper (½ tsp)

- Coarse salt (¾ tsp)
- Grinded cinnamon (½ tsp)
- Grinded cumin (2 tsp)

Direction

Take a large zipper bag and combine pepper, cumin, salt and cinnamon together in it.

Put in chicken and toss to coat.

Now heat oil in a large frying pan and cook chicken in it for about 4 minutes until golden brown.

Toss and cook on the other side for about 2 minutes.

Now take slow cooker and place onion, ginger and onion in it.

Put in chicken and then add tomatoes along with the liquid and raisins.

Cover and cook for about 3 ½ hour on high heat until the chicken is softened.

Serve and enjoy.

Black Bean, Corn And Red Pepper Salad With Lime Cilantro Vinaigrette

Ingredients

- Black beans (15 ounces, rinsed and drained)
- Fresh cooked corn (3 ears) and kernels (2 cup) removed from cob
- 2 Red bell pepper, diced
- 2 garlic cloves, finely minced
- Shallots (2 tbsp), finely minced
- Salt (2 tsp)
- Cayenne pepper (¼ tsp)
- Sugar (2 tbsp)
- Extra virgin olive oil (½ cup + 1 tbsp)
- Lime zest (1 tsp)
- 6 limes, juiced
- Cilantro (½ cup), finely chopped
- Avocados (2 Hass, chopped)

Direction

Combine all the ingredients in a large bowl except avocado and let it stand for about 30 minutes to cool.

Fold in avocado and add to the above mixture.

Serve and enjoy.

Corn Chowder

Ingredients

- 1 onion, finely chopped
- Olive oil (2 tbsp)
- Carrot (1 cup), finely chopped
- Celery (1 cup), finely chopped
- 1 clove of garlic, minced
- Vegetable bouillon (2 cubes)
- Water (2 ½ cups)
- Soy milk (2 cups)
- Corn (2 cups)
- Flour (1 tbsp)
- Garlic powder (1 tsp)
- Dried parsley (1 tsp)
- Black pepper (1 tsp)
- Salt (1 tsp)

Direction

Heat oil in a large frying pan and cook onions and celery in it for about 7 minutes.

Put in garlic and carrots and cook further for about 5 minutes.

Now take a large pot, boil water in it and add bouillon.

When it dissolve completely then add corn and vegetables.

Let it simmer until the vegetables are completely done.

Reduce the heat and then add soymilk.

Stir constantly to become thicken.

Now put in pepper, parsley, salt and garlic powder and stir for about 15 minutes until the desired thickness is obtained.

Serve warm and enjoy.

Dinner Recipes

Roasted Pepper And Cauliflower

Ingredients

- Cheese (4 ounces), crumbled
- Red pepper flakes (¼ tsp)
- Smoked paprika (1 tsp)

- Dried thyme (1 tsp)
- Garlic powder (1 tsp)
- Pepper and salt according to taste
- Heavy cream (½ cup)
- Chicken broth (3 cups)
- 3 medium size green onions, finely diced
- Half head of cauliflower, cut into florets
- 2 red bell peppers, cut into half and remove seeds.
- Oil (2 tbsp)

Direction

Preheat the oven to 400 degrees Fahrenheit.

Remove seeds from pepper, wash and cut into half.

Now broil the pepper for about 15 minutes until blacken.

Place in the container having lid to steam while cooking cauliflower.

Sprinkle with pepper and salt and cook for about half hour.

Peel off the skin of pepper carefully.

Heat diced onion along with 2 tbsp oil in a separate pot and heat well.

Put in seasoning and then add chicken broth along with cauliflower and pepper to the pan.

Cook on low for about 20 minutes.

Put in cream and mix well.

Garnish with thyme and green onion and serve with cheese.

Slow Cooker Buffalo Chicken Soup

Ingredients

- Cream cheese (2 ounces)
- Heavy cream (1 cup)
- Pepper and salt according to taste
- Hot sauce (½ cup)
- Beef broth (3 cups)
- Butter (¼ cup)
- Celery seeds (½ tsp)
- Garlic powder (1 tsp)
- Onion powder (1 tsp)
- 3 chicken thighs, boneless and sliced

Direction

Cut the chicken thighs into small pieces and add to the slow cooker along with all the other ingredients except cream cheese. Cook for about 6 hours on low.

Remove the chicken once done and then shred by using fork.

Put in cream cheese and mix well.

Now put the shredded chicken back to the cooker and mix well.

Flavor it with pepper and salt.

Serve and enjoy.

Spaghetti Squash Lasagna

Ingredients

- Large glass baking dish
- Ground beef (3 pound)
- Cooked spaghetti squash (5 cups)
- Cream cheese (4 cups)
- Hot sauce (1 large jar)

- Mozzarella cheese (30 slices)

Direction

Preheat the oven to 350 degrees Fahrenheit.

Split the spaghetti squash and place it in the baking dish covered with water.

Now place in the oven for about 45-50 minutes until the skin can be forked easily.

As squash cook, start browning meat.

Add sauce over the meat once it is browned and cooked.

Stir thoroughly and let it heat over low heat.

Split the squash gently when cooked.

When ready to arrange lasagna, you must have all the ingredients in reach.

Take a baking dish and place a layer of squash over it.

Top with meat sauce followed by mozzarella slices.

Repeat the same process till end.

But end with mozzarella cheese as a top layer.

Now bake in the oven for about half hour until the cheese turns to golden brown and liquid bubbled out.

Serve hot and enjoy.

Cucumber Sandwich

Ingredients

- Cheese (6 tsp)
- 1 slice meat
- 1 cucumber

Direction

Take the cucumber and cut into longitudinal pieces.

Remove seeds by with the help of spoon.

Spread cheese over one side and place the other side over it. Serve.

Borscht

Ingredients

- Silken tofu (16 ounce)
- Salt (¼ tsp)
- Black pepper (¼ tsp)
- Dried dill weed (2 tbsp)
- Water (4 cups)
- 3 garlic cloves, finely minced
- Olive oil (4 tbsp)
- 1 onion, finely chopped
- 2 stalks of celery, finely chopped
- 2 carrots, finely chopped
- 3 beets including green, diced
- 1 green bell pepper, finely chopped
- Canned whole tomatoes (16 ounce), peeled
- Potatoes (2 quartered)
- Canned tomatoes (½ cup), peeled and diced
- Vegetable broth (2 cups)
- Shredded chard (1 cup)

Direction

Heat about 1 tbsp of oil in a large pan and cook garlic and onion for 5 minutes in it until fragrant.

Heat the remaining oil in a large pot over medium high heat and put in bell pepper, celery, carrots, whole and diced tomatoes, beets, chard potatoes and onion mixture and stir for about 8 minutes until done.

Add broth, water, dill and pepper and let it boil.

Minimize the heat and simmer for about an hour.

Strain half of the beets from the soup and blend until smooth.

Put in tofu and puree again and blend well.

Take a large pot, shift the above mixture to the pot and simmer for about an hour.

Serve and enjoy.

Minestrone

Ingredients

- 1 onion, finely chopped
- Vegetable oil (1 tbsp)
- 2 stalk celery, chopped
- Italian seasoning (2 ½ tsp)

- Black pepper (¼ tsp)
- Salt (¼ tsp)
- Vegetable broth (5 cups)
- Canned Italian style tomato diced (28 ounces)
- 2 carrots, sliced
- 2 sweet potatoes, diced
- Green beans (6 ounces), finely chopped
- 5 cloves of garlic, minced

Direction

Heat oil in a large pot and cook onion, celery, pepper, seasoning and salt in it for about 5 minutes.

Put in tomatoes, garlic, carrots, green beans, sweet potatoes, broth and can juice and mix well and boil.

Reduce the heat and then mix occasionally for about 30 minutes.

Serve and enjoy.

Lentil Soup

Ingredients

- Cayenne pepper (1 pinch)
- Salt (¼ tsp)
- Black pepper (¼ tsp)
- 1 onion, chopped
- Peanut oil (1 tbsp)
- Ginger (1 tbsp), finely minced
- Fenugreek seeds (1 pinch)
- 1 garlic clove, finely chopped
- Dry lentils (1 cup)
- Fresh cilantro (1/3 cup), finely chopped
- Butternut squash (1 cup), peeled, seeded and cubed
- Canned coconut milk (14 ounces)
- Water (2 cups)
- Curry powder (1 tsp)
- Tomato paste (2 tbsp)
- Nutmeg (1 pinch), grounded

Direction

Cook fenugreek seeds, onion, ginger and garlic in a large pot on medium high heat for about 5 minutes.

Put in squash, lentil and cilantro and cook for about 1 minute.

Add coconut oil, salt, pepper, cayenne, nutmeg, curry powder, tomato paste and water and boil.

Then reduce the heat and simmer for about half hour.

Serve.

Fried Eggs With Green Salsa

Ingredients

- Cilantro (½ cup), thinly sliced
- 2 jalapenos, chopped
- Tomatillos (1 cup), chopped
- Salt as needed
- Lime juice (1 cup)
- 3 medium garlic cloves, finely minced
- Tomato (1 cup), chopped
- 2 jalapenos
- Red salsa
- 2 large eggs
- Olive oil (4 tbsp)

Direction

Mix garlic, jalapenos, tomatoes, lime juice and garlic together to make red salsa.

Give it a few high speed pulses until for a chunky mixture.

Shift to the bowl and add cilantro and salt.

Mix ingredients of the green salsa in a blender and give few high speed pulses to make green salsa.

Now Heat oil in a pan and cook eggs in it until the white is set.

Serve with green and red salsa.

Prosciutto-Wrapped Scallops

Ingredients

- Radicchio (2 cups)
- Prosciutto (8 pieces)
- Vinegar (2 tbsp)
- Extra virgin olive oil (3 ounces extra)
- 1 tomato plum
- Belgian evdive (2 cups)
- 8 large sea scallops
- Pepper and salt to taste

- 1 shallot

Direction

Preheat the oven to 400 degrees Fahrenheit.

Take a bowl and cut shallot and tomatoes with olive oil.

Now place shallot and tomato in a baking sheet and bake until browned. Set aside.

Blend shallots, vinegar and tomatoes together and flavor it with pepper and salt.

Add olive oil for emulsification.

Cover scallop with prosciutto.

Heat the remaining oil in a frying pan and cook scallops until done. Set aside.

Put in endive and radicchio and mix for about minutes.

Add the roasted tomato mixture.

Now add radicchio mixture on each plate and used scallop as topping while serving.

Spinach Stuffed Mushrooms

Ingredients

- Tamari (1 tsp)
- Red pepper flakes
- Salt (½ tsp)
- Spinach (¼ cup), chopped
- Nutritional yeast (2 tbsp)
- 2 medium garlic, finely minced
- Olive oil (1 tbsp)
- Black pepper (¼ tsp), grounded
- Basil (2 tbsp)
- Tahini (2 tbsp)
- Firm tofu (7 ounces), drained and crumbled
- Onion (¼ cup), diced
- Tofu-spinach filling
- 8 mushrooms, stems removed
- Water (2 tbsp)
- Tamari (1 tbsp)
- Lemon juice (2 tbsp)

Direction

Mix lemon juice, water and tamari together in a dish and mushrooms.

Soak while preparing filling.

Heat oil in a pan and cook onion and garlic in it for about 3 minutes.

Put in tofu and stir for a while.

Now add red bell pepper, salt, tamari, basil, black pepper and spinach and mix well.

Take away from heat and scoop filling with mushroom caps.

Bake for about 15 minutes before serving.

Salmon Fillet With Cucumber

Ingredients

- Granular sugar substitute (½ tsp)
- Fresh tarragon (1 tsp), finely chopped
- Salmon fillets
- Unsalted butter (2 tbsp)
- Salt (½ tsp)
- Vinegar (2 tsp)
- Olive oil (1 tbsp)
- Black pepper (¼ tsp)
- 2 small cucumbers, seedless

Direction

Take cucumber slices, salt and pepper in a bowl.

Heat oil and butter in frying pan and cook fish in it for about 4 minutes on each side.

Place paper towel on the top to absorb excess oil.

Add cucumber, remaining butter, vinegar, tarragon and sugar and divide them into 4 serving plates.

Top with cucumber and serve.

Chicken Culets With Mustard

Ingredients

- 1 scallion, chopped
- Chicken culets (8 ounces)
- 1 egg
- Crashed black pepper (¾ tsp)
- Mustard (1 ½ tbsp)
- Extra virgin olive oil (6 tbsp)
- Heavy cream (2 tbsp)

- Salt (1 tsp)
- All purpose mix (½ cup)

Direction

Take a deep pot and mix pepper, baking mix and salt.

Beat eggs with heavy cream in a separate bowl and dip chicken culets in it.

Afterward dip in a baking mix.

Heat olive oil in a pan over medium high heat and cook culets in it until golden brown. Set aside.

Discard oil from the pan to another pot and then add heavy cream to the pan.

Let it boil and then cook scallion in it until thickens.

Take away from heat.

Add pepper, mustard and salt and then serve.

Cauli-Tots

Ingredients

- Garlic powder according to taste
- Cheddar cheese (3 ounces), grated
- Pepper and salt according to taste
- Frozen cauliflower (one 12 ounce bag)

Direction

Preheat the oven to 400 degrees Fahrenheit.

Place cauliflower in the microwave for about 6 minutes.

Discard water and let it cool.

Now blend in a food processor until smooth.

In the meanwhile, combine garlic powder, pepper, salt and Cheddar cheese together in a bowl.

Shape cauliflower in 1.5 inch ball and then add to the cheese mixture.

Place the cauli-tots on baking sheet for about 10 minutes before serving.

Roasted Cod With Butter And Garlic Lentil

Ingredients

- 2 garlic cloves, minced
- Pepper and salt according to taste
- Butter (1 tbsp)
- Washed lentils (¼ cup)
- Lemon wedge for garnish
- Olive oil (1tbsp)
- Almond flour (1 tsp)
- Prosciutto (1 tbsp), chopped
- Mustard (1/8 tsp)
- Lemon juice (1 tsp)
- 1 garlic clove, finely minced
- Butter (1 tbsp(, softened
- Skinless cod Fillet (7 ounce)

Direction

Preheat the oven to 450 degrees Fahrenheit.

Take lentils with ¾ cup of water in a medium pot and boil.

Then cook for about 20 minutes.

In the meanwhile stir butter, garlic, mustard, almond flour, prosciutto, pepper and salt together.

Heat olive oil in a frying pan over medium high heat when the lentil is done.

Season cod fillet with pepper and salt and cook for about 4 minutes on each side.

Spoon butter over the fillet and bake in the preheated oven for about 2 minutes until done.

Now take a pan and melt butter in it.

Put in garlic and cook for about 5 minutes until browned.

Add lentil and sauté for 1 minute more.

Now place the lentils in a plate topping with cod fillet and pour sauce over it before serving.

Quinoa And Smoked Tofu Salad

Ingredients

- Fresh mint (½ cup)
- Fresh parsley (½ cup, chopped)
- Grape tomatoes (1 cup, halved)

- Cucumber (1 cup, diced)
- Yellow bell pepper (1 small, diced)
- Baked smoked tofu (1 package or 8 ounces), diced
- Fresh grinded pepper (¼ tsp)
- 3 small garlic cloves, finely minced
- Extra virgin olive oil (3 tbsp)
- Lemon juice (¼ cup)
- Quinoa (1 cup, rinsed)
- Salt (¾ tsp, divided)
- Water (2 cups)

Direction

Take water along with half tsp of salt in saucepan and boil.

Put in quinoa and boil again.

Minimize the heat, cover and cook for about 15-20 minutes.

Then spread on the sheet and let it stand for about 10 minutes to cool.

Now combine the remaining salt with lemon juice, oil garlic and pepper in a large bowl and mix well.

Put in bell pepper tomatoes, mint, parsley, tofu and quinoa.

Toss until well mixed. Serve.

Baked Tortellini

Ingredients

- Cheddar cheese (½ cup, grated)
- Fresh basil (1 tbsp, sliced)
- Mozzarella cheese (1 cup, shredded)
- Cream Cheese (½ cup)
- Hot sauce (2 cups)
- Cheese tortellini (1 pound, frozen)

Direction

Preheat the oven to 210 Degrees Celsius.

Take 2 quarts baking dish and brush with cooking spray.

Cook tortellini according to the procedure in a salted water.

Drain and spread over baking dish.

Take a microwave safe bowl and combine Hot sauce with cream cheese.

Switch microwave to high and cook for about 2 minutes.

Pour the sauce over it and splash with cheese.

Now bake 15 minutes more until the cheese start bubbling and turn to golden.

Top with basil and serve quickly.

Slow Cooker Chicken Dressing

Ingredients

- Margarine (2 tbsp)
- Condensed cream of chicken soup (2 cans about 10.75 ounce)
- Chicken broth (2 cans about 14.5 ounce)
- Sage (2 tsp, dried)
- Ground black pepper (1 tsp)
- Salt (1 tsp)
- 1 small onion, chopped
- 4 large eggs, beaten
- Day old bread (8 slices, torn into small pieces)

- Cornbread (1 pan about 9x9 inches, cooked and crumbled)
- 5 skinless and Boneless chicken breast halves

Direction

Place chicken in a pot covered with water and boil.

After boiling let it stand for about 20 minutes to cool and then cut into small pieces.

Now take slow cooker and combine sage, onion, salt, pepper, chicken broth, chicken soup, eggs, cornbread, bread and chicken in it. Stir well and then spread with margarine.

Cover and cook on low for about 3-4 hours.

Uncover and make it fluffy with a fork.

Let it stand for about 15 minutes to cool before serving.

Slow Cooker Buffalo Brisket

Ingredients

- Water (1 cup)
- Chicken broth (2 cups)
- Pepper and salt according to taste
- Dried basil (1 tsp)
- Garlic (2 tsp, chopped)
- Onion (1 small, chopped)
- 1 buffalo brisket (about 3 pound)
- Olive oil (1 tsp)

Direction

Take slow cooker brush with olive oil and then add buffalo brisket along with garlic, onion and basil.

Flavor it with pepper and salt.

Now add water and chicken broth.

Cover and cook for about 6-8 hours on low.

Serve and enjoy.

Slow Cooker White Chili

Ingredients

- Lime juice (1 tbsp)
- Lemon juice (1 tbsp)
- 2 Green onions, chopped
- Fresh cilantro (¼ cup, chopped)
- 1 large tomato, chopped
- Green chilies (1 can), chopped
- Green salsa (1 can about 7 ounce)
- White corn (1 can about 15.25 ounce)
- Chicken broth (1 can about 14.5 ounce)
- White beans (1 can about 15.5 ounce, drained)
- Cooked chicken breast (2 cups, chopped)

Direction

Combine chicken along with green chilies, green salsa, white beans, white corn, broth, lemon juice, lime juice, green onion, cilantro and tomato in a slow cooker.

Switch slow cooker to low heat and cook for about an hour until tender.

Serve and enjoy.

Main Dishes

Asparagus And Chipotle Mayonnaise

Ingredients

- Mayonnaise (½ cup)
- 1 chipotle chili
- Asparagus (2 pounds)

Direction

Discard the ends of asparagus and place in a microwaveable casserole.

Add few tbsp of water to the casserole and then cover with plastic wrap.

Cook for about 5 minutes.

Combine mayonnaise, chipotle and a teaspoon of sauce in a blender and blend until smooth.

Serve asparagus with sauce and enjoy.

Creamed Spinach

Ingredients

- Butter (3 tbsp)
- Cream cheese (2 tbsp)
- Frozen chopped spinach (10 ounces)
- Pepper and salt according to taste

Direction

Nuke spinach in a bowl for about 8 minutes.

Stir and nuke for 1 minute more and then drain.

Shift spinach to the bowl and add butter and cream cheese.

Stir both until melt fully and incorporate evenly to form a smooth sauce.

Add pepper and salt and divide them into portions while serving.

Chicken Curry

Ingredients

- 5 sprigs cilantro

- Kashmiri mirch (½ tsp)
- Ground red chili (½ tsp)
- Fresh ground pepper (1 tsp)
- Paprika (½ tsp)
- Garam masala (1 tsp)
- Salt (1 tsp)
- Garlic paste (1 ½ tsp)
- Coriander powder (1 tsp)
- Coconut oil (2 tsp)
- Garlic paste (1 ½ tsp)
- Butter (4 tbsp)
- Olive oil (1 tbsp)
- Crushed tomatoes (1 cup)
- Heavy cream (½ cup)
- Paneer packet (7 ounce)
- Water (1 cup)
- Chicken thighs (3 pound)

Direction

Preheat the oven to 375 Degrees Fahrenheit.

Rub chicken thighs with olive oil and then add pepper and salt according to taste.

Take cooking sheet, place chicken thighs on it and bake for about 25 minutes.

Cut paneer into small pieces and set them aside.

Heat olive oil with butter in a preheated pan and wait until turns to brown.

Put in paste, ginger and garlic and sauté for about 2 minutes.

Add garam masala, salt, red chili powder, coriander powder and paprika.

Blend them well and simmer until oil shows on the top.

Blend paneer, slowly add water and simmer for about 5 minutes.

Discard the chicken when done and separate from bones.

Dip in a sauce and stir well.

Now simmer for about 5 minutes and splash with cilantro before serving.

Ginger Beef

Ingredients

- Ground ginger (1 tsp)
- Vinegar (4 tbsp)
- 1 garlic clove, crashed
- 2 small tomatoes, diced
- Olive oil (1 tbsp)
- Pepper and salt according to taste
- 1 small onion, diced
- 2 sirloin steak cut into strips

Direction

Heat oil in a pan and fry steak in it until brown.

Add garlic, tomatoes and onions and cook for few minutes until done.

Combine vinegar, ginger salt and pepper in a bowl and then add to the pan.

Cover the pan and simmer until most of the liquid evaporates.

Chicken Salad

Ingredients

- Low sodium beef (1 piece)
- Chili sauce (1 tbsp)
- Half chicken breast
- Half large avocado
- Baby spinach (2 cups)
- Oil for frying

Direction

Heat oil in a saucepan and cook beef in it until crispy and golden brown.

Cut the chicken breast into 2 equal parts while cooking.

In the meanwhile slice avocado into small pieces.

Shift the mixture to the bowl and top with chili sauce while serving.

Beef Scramble And Egg Whites

Ingredients

- 2 Italian tomatoes
- Pepper and salt to taste

- 4 small tomatoes
- Red pepper (½ cup)
- 8 egg whites
- Baby spinach (2 cups)
- Extra ground beef (1 pound)

Direction

Take a pan spray with olive oil and heat over medium high heat.

Cut the beef into small pieces and cook in the oil until golden brown. Set aside.

Beat Eggs and pour the whiter part over cooked meat.

Sauté with spinach, pepper, red basil and tomatoes and then serve.

Fried Chicken

Ingredients

- Water (¼ cup)
- Half ¾ inch deep hot oil
- 2 large eggs

- Heavy cream (¼ cup)
- Cheddar cheese (½ cup)
- Coarse black pepper (1/8 tsp)
- Salt (1 tsp)
- Onion powder (½ tsp)
- Crushed beef rinds (1 cup)
- Oat fiber (1 tbsp)
- Plain whey protein (¾ cup)

Direction

Take a plastic bag, combine all the ingredients in it and mix well.

Now take a bowl and mix eggs, cream and water together.

Now add chopped chicken to the mixture and coat them well.

Season each piece of chopped chicken with flour after removing from the bowl.

Heat oil in a pan and cook chicken piece one by one from both sides until golden brown.

Serve.

Baked Salmon

Ingredients

- 2 salmon fillets
- Lemon juice (1 tbsp)
- Fresh parsley (1 tbsp), chopped
- Salt (1 tsp)
- Grounded black pepper (1 tsp)
- Olive oil (6 tbsp)
- Dried basil (1 tsp)
- 2 clove garlic, finely minced

Direction

Mix garlic, salt, pepper, parsley, lemon juice and olive oil together to form marinade.

Now take a pan and put the fillets in it.

Spread the marinade over the fillets and chill in the refrigerator for about an hour.

Preheat the oven to 375 degrees Fahrenheit.

Take aluminum foil and roll the fillets in it.

Spread with marinade and then seal.

Shift the fillets to the glass plate and then put in the oven until they can produce flakes.

Serve and enjoy.

Curried pecans

Ingredients

- Onion powder (½ tsp)
- Pecans (8 ounces)
- Garlic powder (¼ tsp)
- Coconut oil (3 tbsp)
- Salt according to taste

Direction

Preheat the oven to 350 degrees Fahrenheit.

Melt coconut oil in a pan and add seasoning in it.

Mix the seasoning and then put in pecans.

Mix again after adding pecans until coated well.

Now roast for about 5 minutes and then again mix.

Now roast further for 5 minutes and then allow it to cool.

Add salt according to taste and then divide them into portions before serving.

Pecans

Ingredients

- Pecans (2 cups), halved
- Butter (3 tbsp)
- Salt as needed

Direction

Preheat the oven to 350 degrees Fahrenheit.

Melt butter in a roasting pan and add pecans.

Mix thoroughly until the pecans is uniformly coated.

Mix again after 4 minutes and then roast in the oven for about 5 minutes.

Now remove from the oven, add salt and let it cool for some time before serving.

Divide into portions while serving.

Conclusion

It is my sincere hope that you might have liked all the recipes which have been mentioned in the book and once again thank you for getting this book and experimenting with the recipes.

About The Author

Tamara Henderson is born with the vision to promote *Medterranean Diet* among the masses. The author has written several research papers on the topic. She has served as an instructor promoting various cultural arts in University of San Francisco. She is currently living with his spouse in Texas.

www.ingramcontent.com/pod-product-compliance
Lightning Source LLC
LaVergne TN
LVHW011950070526
838202LV00054B/4872